ULTRA PROCESSED FOOD:

the health risks of food additives

LORRAINE F. FELICIANO

DISCLAIMER

TABLE OF CONTENT

Contents

INTRODUCTION

UNDERSTANDING ULTRA-PROCESSED FOODS

Have you ever wondered what's truly in the food you consume every day? In a society where convenience frequently outweighs nutrition, it's vital to take a deeper look at what we eat. Let's begin on a trip to solve the secrets underlying the foods that dominate our contemporary diet the ultra-processed meals.

The fast-paced scenario

Imagine this scenario: You're hurrying to work, your stomach is grumbling, and you need a quick meal. The answer? an apparently harmless cereal bar. It offers ease, flavor, and a touch of energy to launch your day. But have you ever examined what's lying beneath that wrapper? The elements mentioned may read like a scientific experiment, and in many respects, they are. Your handy breakfast bar undoubtedly falls into the category of ultra-processed meals. In the rush and bustle of contemporary life, we frequently grab for these ultra-convenient and easily accessible food items.

However, it's time to halt and ponder their ramifications. These items have grown widespread in our diets, lining grocery store shelves, filling vending machines, and finding their way into our homes. The emergence of ultra-processed meals matches a fast-paced culture that prizes ease and quickness. But what do we compromise in the name of convenience?

The answers may be more crucial than you believe.

What are ultra-processed foods?

Before we dig further into the realm of ultra-processed foods, let's start by defining what they are. These foods are distant from their natural nature. They undergo substantial processing, frequently comprising many rounds of industrial operations, which add compounds that may not resemble ordinary kitchen components.

Ultra-processed foods are those industrial formulations often generated from ingredients taken from entire foods (such as oils, lipids, sugar, starch, and proteins) with little or no whole foods. They frequently include additives such as taste enhancers, food coloring, emulsifiers, and other cosmetic components.

With such intricate compositions, their objective is to be very lucrative, convenient, hyper-palatable, and appealing. Understanding ultra-processed foods is crucial since they have become a fundamental element of the contemporary diet.

Many of us eat these things regularly, sometimes without even realizing it. They've invaded the food business and, in turn, our lives, altering our diets, our health, and our perception of what it means to eat.

The Purpose of This Book

This book intends to shine a light on ultra-processed foods, analyzing their prevalence in our diets, their consequences on our health, and the choices we make as consumers. We'll dig into the science behind these meals, studying the influence of their intake on different elements of well-being. In our trip through this book, we will explore issues such as diet, health effects, genetics, and alternative alternatives. We'll cover how food processing affects what we consume, how we perceive food, and the impact on our bodies.

Navigating the chapters

To give you a sense of what to anticipate, let's quickly describe the chapters of this book:

Chapter 1: What Are Ultra-Processed Foods? In this chapter, we'll establish the groundwork by defining the phrase "ultra-processed foods." We'll investigate how these meals are created and what distinguishes them from other types.

Chapter 2: The Impact of Ultra-Processed Foods on Health We'll go into the ramifications of ingesting ultra-processed foods, their effect on the body, and their position in the global health scene.

Chapter 3: The Science Behind Ultra-Processed Foods Get ready to learn about the intricate and intriguing world of food processing. We'll examine the strategies employed to make these items and the science behind them.

Chapter 4: The Hidden Dangers: Ingredients and Additives Here, we'll investigate the components and additives often found in ultra-processed meals. We'll also dig into the possible health dangers linked to these additions.

Chapter 5: Nutrition and Ultra-Processed Foods We'll explore the nutritional features of ultra-processed foods, comparing them to complete, unprocessed meals. What are the distinctions, and how do they affect our diets?

Chapter 6: Genetics and Weight: Exploring the Connection Genetics plays a part in our body's reaction to varied diets. In this chapter, we'll study the connection between genetics and weight gain in the context of ultra-processed meals.

Chapter 7: Unprocessed Food Alternatives When it comes to eating healthier food, there are many choices available. We'll investigate unprocessed food choices, giving insights into adding whole, natural foods to your diet.

Chapter 8: Health Consequences of Unhealthy Eating What happens when we don't pay attention to our nutritional choices? We'll cover the repercussions of a bad diet, touching on blood pressure, allergies, skin health, and the risk of illnesses like type 2 diabetes.

Chapter 9: Nutrition for Active Lifestyles For individuals living busy lifestyles or indulging in sports, it's necessary to nourish the body sufficiently. In this chapter, we'll look into the dietary demands of those with busy lives.

Chapter 10: Identifying and Avoiding Ultra-Processed Foods We'll complete our trip by offering practical tips on detecting ultra-processed foods and making educated choices for a better diet.

This book isn't simply about awareness; it's about empowerment. It's about choosing decisions that positively influence our health and well-being. So, let's go on this adventure of research and discovery as we uncover the complexity and secrets of ultra-processed meals. In the pages that follow, you'll discover insights, guidance, and practical techniques to help you make educated choices about your diet and, in turn, your life.

CHAPTER 2

WHAT ARE ULTRA-PROCESSED FOODS

In a world where the number of food options may be bewildering, it's vital to understand the varied degrees of food processing and their influence on our health. We'll start our adventure by investigating the phrase "ultra-processed foods" and solving the secrets of these omnipresent, modern-day dietary companions.

The Spectrum of Food Processing

To grasp ultra-processed meals, it's vital to differentiate between distinct forms of food processing. Food processing isn't necessarily bad; it's the degree and motivation behind the processing that count.

Here's a breakdown:

Unprocessed Foods: Unprocessed foods are the purest source of nourishment. They consist of entire, natural components that have undergone minimal to no modifications before reaching your plate. Think fresh fruits and vegetables, healthy grains, and lean meats. These foods are at the heart of a healthy diet.

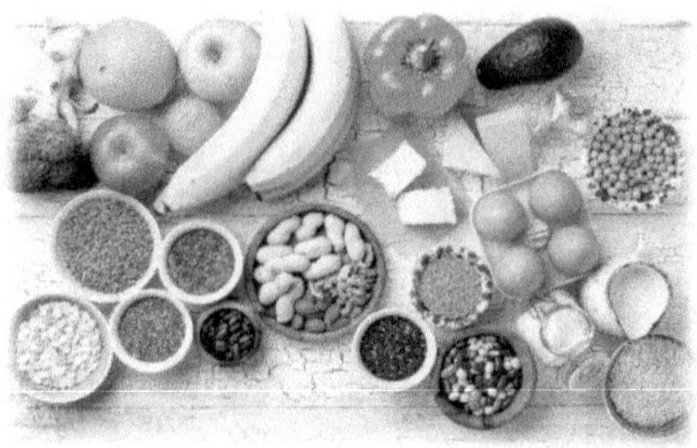

Minimally processed foods:

Minimally processed foods are the bridge between unprocessed and processed meals. While they've had some degree of processing, it's often for preservation or improvement without compromising their basic nutritional content. For example, bagged spinach, roasted almonds, and canned beans

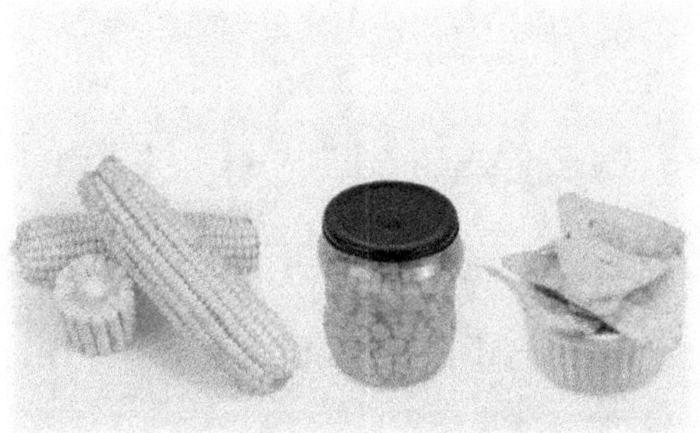

Processed Foods: Processed foods

undergo more substantial modifications, frequently requiring heating, grinding, or the inclusion of preservatives. These dishes may include multiple components, yet they still maintain some sort of similarity to their original condition. Think of spaghetti, cheese, or canned tomato sauce.

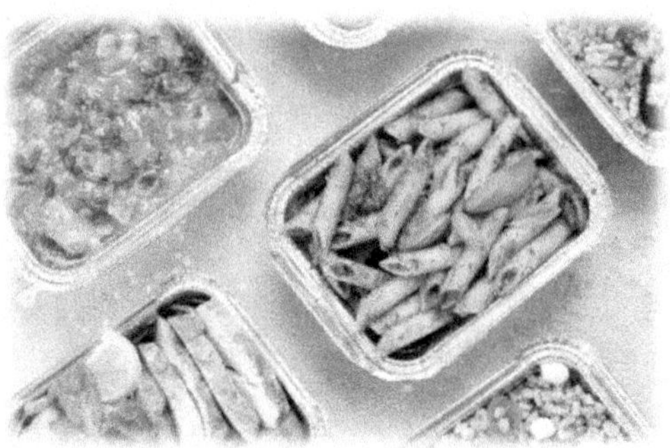

Ultra-Processed Foods: Ultra-processed foods, our core emphasis, represent the extreme end of the processing continuum. They undergo several industrial procedures that alter the constituents into formulations far from their natural condition. These meals frequently include chemicals, including preservatives, artificial flavors, and sweeteners. They bear scant similarity to entire foods.

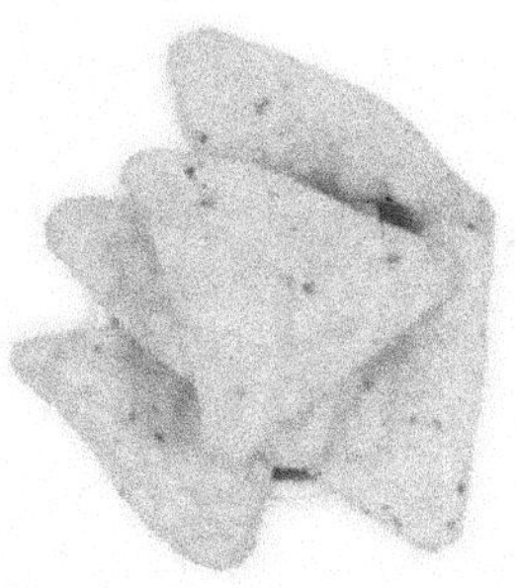

Examples of ultra-processed foods are prevalent and may include sugary cereals, soft drinks, packaged snacks, and fast food products. These items dominate the aisles of supermarkets and convenience shops, luring customers with their convenience and frequently hyper-palatable tastes.

Unraveling the Mystery: What Sets Ultra-Processed Foods Apart?

The primary differentiators between ultra-processed meals and their less-processed alternatives include:

1. Ingredient Complexity: Ultra-processed meals consist of multiple ingredients, typically containing artificial chemicals, colorings, and taste enhancers. You'll discover vast lists of compounds, many of which can be unidentifiable.

2. Industrial Formulation: The manufacture of ultra-processed meals includes complex industrial procedures. These foods are manufactured using ingredients taken from entire foods, such as oils, lipids, sugar, starch, and proteins. These components undergo many steps of processing to form the final product.

3. Reduced entire foods: ultra-processed foods include little to no entire foods. Unlike processed meals like canned veggies or dry pasta, ultra-processed foods depend on extra additives to produce a pleasing, sometimes addictive product.

Common Misconceptions About Processed Foods

As we explore the realm of ultra-processed meals, it's necessary to dispel certain myths regarding processed foods in general. Understanding these differences may lead to smarter choices and a more educated approach to your food.

1. Processing Is Always Harmful: Processing food isn't necessarily harmful. In truth, some amount of processing is essential to making some foods safe, tasty, and convenient. For example, pasteurization ensures milk is safe to consume, while freezing protects nutrients in fruits and vegetables.

2. All Processed Foods Are Unhealthy: Not all processed foods should be criticized. Many minimally processed meals are healthy and provide convenience without compromising health. For example, plain yogurt, frozen veggies, and whole-grain bread come into this category.

3. You Should Eliminate All Processed Foods: Aiming to eliminate all processed foods from your diet may not be realistic or required. It's about making educated decisions. Some processed foods are part of a balanced diet, but the key is to concentrate on those that preserve their nutritional content.

By differentiating between these categories and correcting myths, we build the framework for a more thorough knowledge of ultra-processed foods. In the chapters that follow, we'll dig further into their influence on health and examine the choices we can make to create a better connection with the foods we consume.

CHAPTER 3

THE SCIENCE BEHIND ULTRA-PROCESSED FOODS

As we venture farther into the domain of ultra-processed foods, it's vital to peel back the layers of science and technology that drive these pervasive dietary choices. Understanding the complicated procedures employed in making these items and the function of ingredients, additives, and chemical processes is important in unraveling the attractiveness of ultra-processed meals.

The Alchemy of Food Processing

At first glance, the preparation of ultra-processed meals would seem to be a complicated type of culinary alchemy. However, these items depend on a complex combination of science, technology, and invention to create their distinctive traits. Let's investigate some of the main aspects that turn raw materials into the appealing, hyper-palatable delicacies we see on shop shelves.

Ingredients: The Building Blocks

Ingredients are the basis of any culinary product. When it comes to ultra-processed meals, they generally employ a combination of fundamental components as a starting point.

These components include:

Refined sugars: are often used to increase sweetness and palatability.

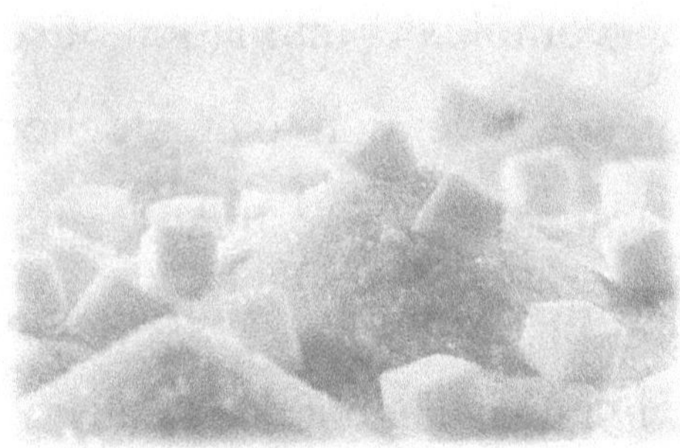

Processed fats and oils: are frequently incorporated for texture and mouthfeel.

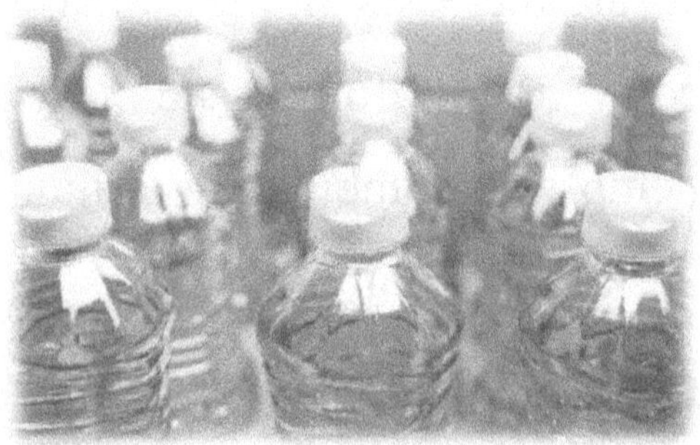

Modified Starches: Used to enhance texture and uniformity.

Artificial Flavorings and Sweeteners: Added to produce tempting flavor characteristics.

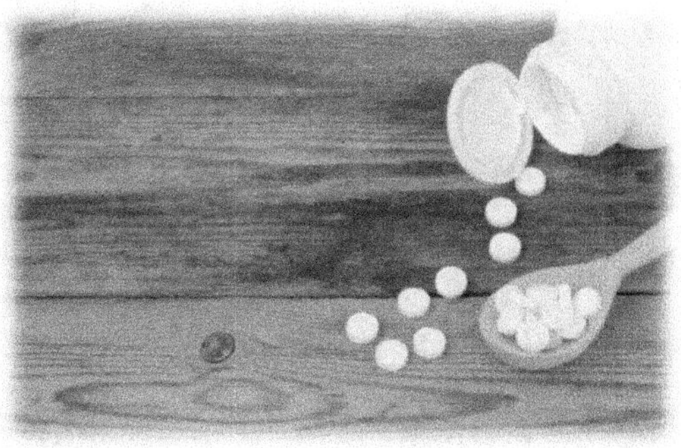

Preservatives: extend shelf life and prevent spoilage.

Artificial colors: enhance visual attractiveness.

These components, although not intrinsically dangerous in moderation, play a crucial role in making ultra-processed meals attractive. It's the mix and management of these components that produce the unique taste, texture, and shelf-stability of such items.

Additives: The secret sauce

In the realm of ultra-processed meals, additives are the secret sauce. They're the unsung heroes that change and intensify the sensory experience. Here are some typical additions you could encounter:

Monosodium glutamate (MSG): Known for its flavor-enhancing characteristics, MSG adds a savory taste, frequently characterized as umami.

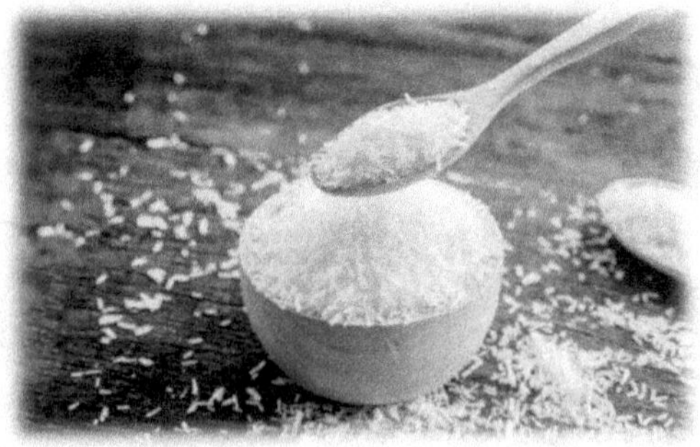

High-Fructose Corn Syrup (HFCS): A sweetening compound that's cheaper and sweeter than ordinary sugar, contributing to the excessive sweetness of many ultra-processed goods.

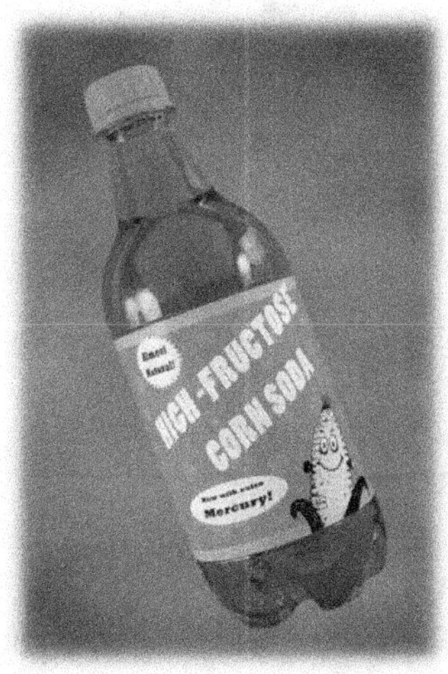

Emulsifiers: These substances enhance the stability and texture of processed meals, preventing components from separating.

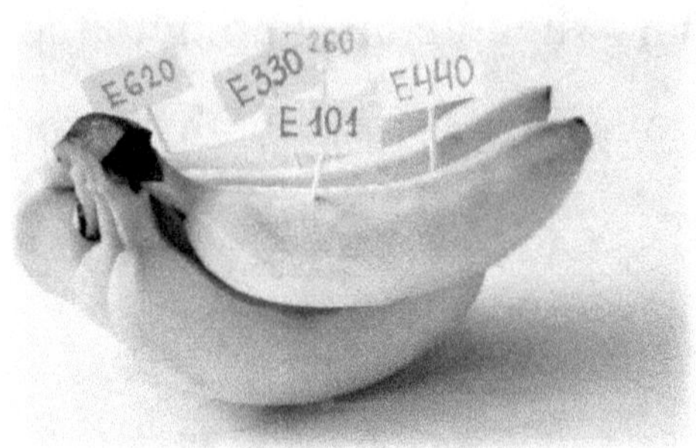

Texturizers: are used to generate the appropriate mouthfeel, from the crispness of potato chips to the smoothness of a chocolate bar.

Thickeners: These ingredients guarantee that processed meals have the correct consistency.

As you can see, these additives aren't always dangerous by themselves. However, it's their ubiquitous usage in ultra-processed meals that causes problems. They're purposefully deployed to make delicacies that are virtually impossible to refuse.

Chemical Processes: The Transformation

The chemical procedures involved in generating ultra-processed meals are key to their attractiveness.

While this can seem frightening, it's vital to understand that processing can take numerous forms. Some typical ways include:

Extrusion: Used to generate the distinctive forms and textures of many processed delicacies, including chips and puffed cereals.

Hydrogenation: is a procedure that hardens liquid fats, giving ultra-processed foods a more acceptable texture and shelf stability.

Flavor Enhancement: Chemicals are employed to replicate natural flavors, giving a strong taste sensation.

Dehydration: Removing moisture from food is a preservation strategy, but it also boosts the concentration of tastes.

Understanding these processes gives vital insight into why ultra-processed foods may be so addicting. They're created to deliver a powerful sensory experience that keeps you wanting for more.

The Power of Palatability

Palatability, or the sensory pleasure obtained from eating, is one of the distinguishing qualities of ultra-processed meals. These items are painstakingly developed to be as attractive as possible to our senses.

They typically mix the senses of sweetness, saltiness, and richness, producing an appealing trifecta. These meals are meant to activate the pleasure regions in our brain, leading to cravings and an almost instinctive want for more.

Understanding the physics underlying these feelings is vital, as it allows us to make better educated decisions and ask if the attraction is worth the possible implications for our health.

Visualizing the journey

To help in appreciating the intricate science underlying ultra-processed meals, let's explore a simple graphic representation:

Ingredients: These are the building blocks of ultra-processed meals, supplying the core components.

Additives: Think of them as the enhancers that make the sensory experience pop, comparable to seasoning in a dish.

Chemical Processes: These reflect the numerous cooking, combining, and changing procedures utilized in food processing.

Palatability: Imagine a sensory explosion when tastes, textures, and scents merge together to produce a joyful, even irresistible experience.

As we go further into the pages of this chapter, recall this visual framework. It will help you uncover the layers of intricacy that make ultra-processed meals such a ubiquitous and compelling presence in our lives. In the chapters that follow, we'll investigate the influence of these foods on our health and well-being and learn methods to navigate a world saturated with enticing, ultra-processed alternatives.

CHAPTER 4

THE HIDDEN DANGERS: INGREDIENTS AND ADDICTIVES

In our quest to uncover the mysteries behind ultra-processed meals, we must gaze into the core of these products the ingredients and additives that contribute to their peculiar aromas, textures, and lifespan. It's here, amid the chemical compounds and preservatives, that we unearth hidden risks.

The Chemistry of Flavor Enhancement

Ultra-processed foods are recognized for their amazing flavor and are frequently regarded as addicting. This taste profile is not an accident;

it's the product of a carefully constructed mix of chemicals and substances meant to capture your senses.

Monosodium Glutamate (MSG): The Umami Enigma

Let's begin with a notable star in the world of additives monosodium glutamate, or MSG. MSG is a flavor enhancer responsible for providing the delicious and rich taste known as umami. It's present in various ultra-processed foods, from savory snacks to ready-made dinners.

MSG was initially extracted from seaweed soup in Japan more than a century ago, and since then, it's been a major element in generating the powerful, delicious flavor that's virtually irresistible. But what's the downside?

Several studies have highlighted concerns about the possible health consequences of MSG, including headaches, perspiration, and a feeling frequently referred to as "Chinese restaurant syndrome." However, these effects are rarely regularly seen and are often minor. The U.S. Food and Drug Administration (FDA) deems MSG safe when ingested in moderation. It's vital to be aware of the quantity you eat, since large quantities might possibly lead to unpleasant responses.

High-Fructose Corn Syrup (HFCS):

The Sweet Menace High-fructose corn syrup (HFCS) is a widely used sweetening component in ultra-processed foods. It's cheaper and sweeter than regular sugar, which makes it a favored option for producers. You'll find it in soft drinks, candies, baked products, and several other sweet delicacies.

The difficulty with HFCS resides in its possible connection to obesity and numerous associated health disorders. Consuming excessive quantities of added sugars, particularly in the form of HFCS, is connected to weight gain, insulin resistance, and metabolic syndrome. It's crucial to be cautious of your sugar consumption, particularly when eating foods containing HFCS.

The alarming truth about preservatives

Preservatives are another type of chemical typically found in ultra-processed foods. Their major function is to increase the product's shelf life, ensuring it stays in a pleasant state for a longer duration. But these compounds come with their own set of hazards.

Artificial Colors: Appealing but Risky

Artificial colors are applied to improve the visual attractiveness of ultra-processed meals. Think about vividly colored candy, drinks, and varied foods. While these brilliant colors could be visually alluring, there are still concerns regarding their safety.

The FDA has authorized various artificial colors; however, some research reveals a possible relationship between some artificial colorings and hyperactivity in youngsters. While further study is required to corroborate these results, it's advisable to eat vivid, artificially colored foods in moderation, particularly for youngsters.

Sulfites: hidden troublemakers

Sulfites are utilized as preservatives in several ultra-processed foods, notably dried fruits, wine, and some processed meats. These molecules help avoid rotting and discoloration but may represent dangers to people sensitive to sulfites. Sulfite sensitivity may lead to allergic symptoms, including skin rashes, hives, and breathing problems.

While not everyone is sensitive to sulfites, it's crucial to be aware of their existence in foods if you encounter allergic reactions.

The Power of Knowledge

Understanding the chemicals and additives in ultra-processed meals empowers us with the capacity to make educated decisions. While certain additives, like MSG, have a relatively moderate influence on health when ingested in moderation, others, such as HFCS and some artificial colors, pose more serious concerns.

When we stand back and study the chemicals and additives included in these meals, it becomes clear that our decisions have a direct influence on our health and well-being. Armed with information, we may make mindful judgments about the ultra-processed foods we eat, enabling us to relish the tastes we like while limiting any health hazards.

In the chapters that follow, we'll look further into the larger repercussions of eating ultra-processed meals. From studying their impact on the human body to examining techniques for lessening our dependency on them, we're beginning a journey toward a healthier and more conscious approach to eating.

CHAPTER 5

NUTRITION AND ULTRA-PROCESSED FOODS

In the era of convenience, our food choices have undergone a tremendous shift. A significant share of our meals consist of ultra-processed foods, luring us with their convenience and seductive tastes. But what do these foods provide in terms of nutrition? In this chapter, we look into the nutritional value of ultra-processed foods, comparing them to entire, unprocessed alternatives.

The Nutrition Divide

When it comes to nutrition, it's crucial to know that not all foods are created equal. The gap between whole, unprocessed meals and their ultra-processed alternatives is obvious, affecting not just our health but also our total well-being.

Whole, unprocessed foods

Whole, unprocessed foods, such as fruits, vegetables, whole grains, lean meats, and legumes, are the cornerstones of a healthy diet. They are rich with important vitamins, minerals, fiber, and antioxidants that promote healthy health. The charm of entire foods resides in their natural nature.

They provide genuine, unmodified nutrients, free from additions, preservatives, and artificial components. When we eat entire meals, we provide our bodies with the nutrients required for development, healing, and maintenance. These meals have a favorable influence on our energy levels, immune system, and general vitality.

Ultra-Processed Foods

On the opposite end of the range, we have ultra-processed foods. These items frequently provide little or no nutritional value when compared to entire foods. While they may give a rapid energy boost and provide robust tastes, they fall short in supplying important nutrients.

A big worry with ultra-processed meals is the excessive concentration of added sugars, harmful fats, and high levels of salt.

These components lead to an increased risk of chronic health conditions, including obesity, heart disease, and type 2 diabetes. In addition to their poor nutritional content, ultra-processed foods are frequently engineered to be hyper-palatable. This implies they're purposefully engineered to be incredibly delectable, making it simple to overconsume calories without feeling satisfied.

Consequences of an Ultra-Processed Diet

The disadvantages of a diet primarily dependent on ultra-processed foods extend beyond basic nutritional inadequacies. These foods may contribute to a variety of health concerns, many of which are on the increase in communities where ultra-processed diets are common.

Nutrient Deficiencies: One of the most apparent implications of a diet predominantly focused on ultra-processed foods is the possibility of nutritional shortages. While these items frequently provide a lot of empty calories, they lack the vital vitamins and minerals required for a well-rounded diet.

The lack of important nutrients may result in deficits that harm our health in many ways. For example, the absence of dietary fiber, often present in whole foods, may contribute to digestive difficulties and an increased risk of colon cancer. The lack of antioxidants, which are plentiful in fresh fruits and vegetables, might lead to oxidative stress and chronic illnesses.

Weight gain and obesity: Weight control is a vital element of health, and ultra-processed meals typically lead to weight gain and obesity. Their high calorie density, coupled with the fact that they don't produce fullness, makes it easy to overeat. Excess calorie intake, especially when it becomes a habit, leads to weight gain.

Moreover, the high sugar content in many ultra-processed meals, frequently in the form of high-fructose corn syrup, plays a role in the development of insulin resistance and metabolic syndrome. These disorders raise the risk of type 2 diabetes and heart disease.

Chronic health issues: Ultra-processed meals are closely connected to the development of chronic health conditions, including heart disease, hypertension, and type 2 diabetes. The excessive consumption of harmful fats and added sugars exerts great stress on our cardiovascular system and may lead to atherosclerosis, increased blood pressure, and insulin resistance.

Furthermore, evidence reveals a probable relationship between a diet high in ultra-processed foods and some malignancies, notably those of the colon and rectum.

Scientific Findings on Ultra-Processed Food Nutrition: Scientific studies give a lot of data on the nutritional features of ultra-processed meals and their health effects. Researchers have researched the dietary habits of people and evaluated the impact of ingesting various goods.

The results underline the necessity of minimizing our dependence on ultra-processed meals. For instance, research published in the journal Nutrients indicated that people with a high intake of ultra-processed foods are likely to have diets deficient in fiber, vitamins, and minerals.

This eating pattern relates to shortages of important nutrients. Another study, published in the journal JAMA Internal Medicine, evaluated the relationship between ultra-processed food intake and the risk of cardiovascular disease. The findings indicated a clear relationship between a larger consumption of these goods and a greater chance of heart-related disorders.

As the scientific data continues to grow, it's evident that our dietary choices have a substantial impact on determining our health. Reducing our consumption of ultra-processed meals and boosting our intake of full, unprocessed choices is a proactive step toward enhancing our nutritional well-being. In the next chapters, we'll further analyze the consequences of an ultra-processed diet on particular elements of health, highlighting the necessity of making thoughtful choices when it comes to the foods we eat.

CHAPTER 6

GENETICS AND WEIGHT: EXPLORING THE CONNECTION

The relationship between heredity and weight has long been a topic of curiosity and scientific research. In this chapter, we look into the intricate link between our genetic makeup and body composition, attempting to identify how our genes impact our weight.

The Genetic Blueprint

Each of us carries a unique genetic blueprint, a collection of instructions contained in our DNA that plays a key role in defining our physical features. These genetic instructions control everything from our height and eye color to more sophisticated features like metabolism and body fat distribution.

<u>Genetics and body composition</u>

The genetic effect on human body composition, including body weight and fat distribution, is complicated. Various genetic variables come into play:

1. Metabolism: Our genes largely affect the pace at which we burn calories and turn food into energy. A quick metabolism helps some people consume more without gaining weight, whereas a slower metabolism might contribute to easy weight gain.

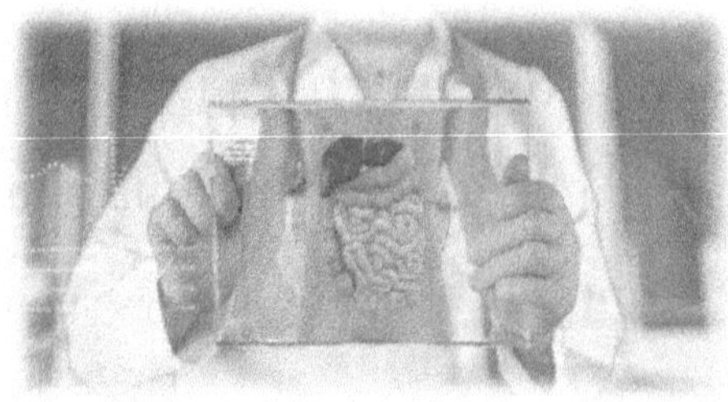

2. Fat Storage: Genetics also impact where our bodies store fat. Some people are genetically prone to retaining fat in their abdominal region, which is connected with a greater risk of health concerns, including heart disease and type 2 diabetes.

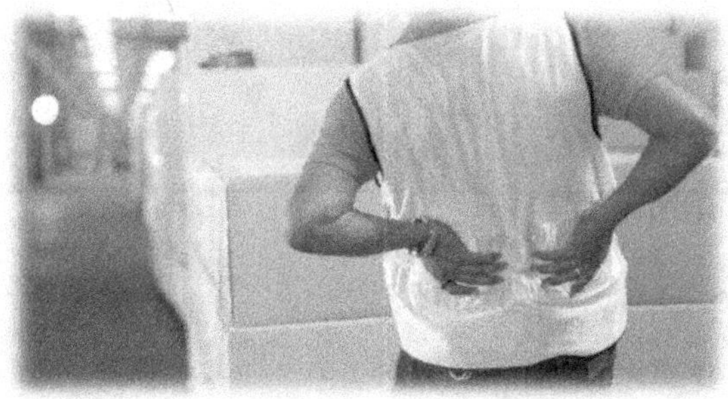

3. Appetite Regulation: Our genetic composition may affect how our bodies manage appetite and fullness. Some genes control the generation of hunger hormones, while others alter our brain's reaction to food signals and desires.

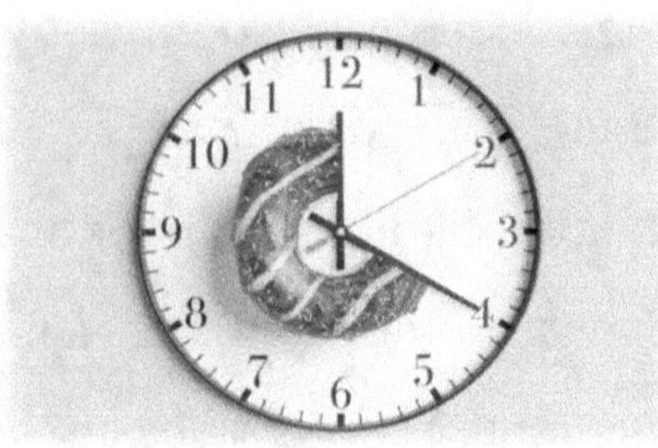

4. Insulin Sensitivity: Genetic factors may lead to differences in insulin sensitivity. This changes how our bodies control blood sugar, altering weight management and the likelihood of developing type 2 diabetes.

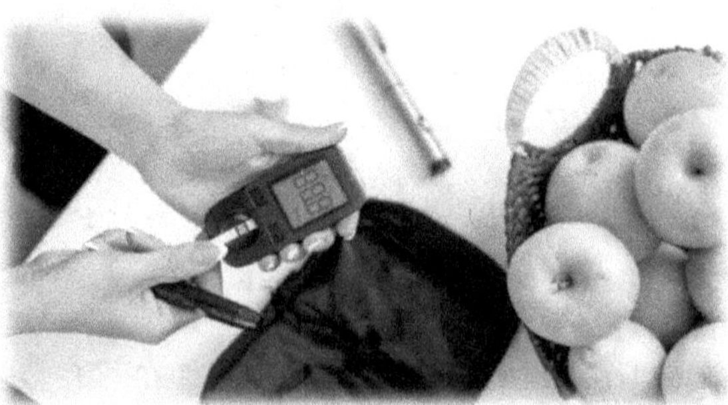

Genes and Diet Response

One of the intriguing features of genetics is its involvement in shaping our reactions to varied diets and food kinds. Some people may find it easier to lose weight on a low-carb diet, while others could have greater success with a low-fat or balanced diet.

This phenomenon is frequently referred to as "nutrigenetics." Research in the subject of nutrigenetics is always advancing. Scientists are aiming to uncover particular genes that have a role in food response. For example, research published in the journal Diabetologia evaluated the effect of the FTO gene on weight control.

The FTO gene is connected with an increased risk of obesity, and the research indicated that people with certain mutations of this gene may be more susceptible to certain dietary treatments. The relationship between heredity and weight also extends to our capacity to taste and prefer different tastes. For instance, mutations in the TAS2R38 gene might impact a person's sensitivity to bitter tastes, thereby influencing their dietary choices.

Case Studies and Research Findings

The role of heredity in weight becomes evident when we analyze case studies and research data. By researching particular genetic variants and their influence on people, scientists have made considerable gains in understanding the genetic components of obesity and body weight. The

Pima Indians

One of the most interesting case studies includes the Pima Indians, a group with a high rate of obesity and type 2 diabetes. Researchers determined that a distinct genetic mutation predisposes this group to obesity when exposed to a Westernized diet. This genetic vulnerability illustrates the extensive interaction between genes and the environment in determining weight.

The Fat Mass and Obesity-Associated (FTO) Gene

The FTO gene, as indicated before, has been the focus of substantial investigation. Scientists have found particular variants of the FTO gene linked with an increased risk of obesity. This gene is involved in the control of appetite and energy expenditure. Understanding how it acts gives information on the genetic variables regulating weight.

The Role of Leptin

Leptin is a hormone that plays a critical role in controlling hunger and body weight. Researchers have revealed that some genetic abnormalities might lead to leptin resistance, limiting the body's capacity to perceive fullness. This syndrome may lead to overeating and weight gain, even when calorie intake is high.

The Complex Interaction

It's crucial to remember that although genetics obviously impact our weight, they don't dictate our destiny. The relationship between genetics and lifestyle variables is complicated. While some people may have genetic predispositions that make weight control more problematic, lifestyle choices, such as nutrition and physical exercise, may dramatically affect the result. In the following chapter, we'll look into how lifestyle variables and genetics interact and how people may negotiate these effects to attain their weight management objectives.

CHAPTER 7

<u>UNPROCESSED FOOD ALTERNATIVES</u>

Transitioning from a diet heavy on ultra-processed foods to one focused on full, unprocessed components may seem like a daunting undertaking. However, this chapter attempts to make this change more accessible and practical by providing you with a toolset of unprocessed food choices and inspired recipes to jumpstart your journey.

<u>A Step Towards Wholesome Eating</u>

Understanding the influence of ultra-processed meals on our health and well-being is the first step towards adopting unprocessed alternatives.

As you've studied in the preceding chapters, the chemicals, additives, and nutritional content of ultra-processed foods create considerable issues. The good news is that making the move to unprocessed foods doesn't have to be a radical or overwhelming adjustment; it can be a gradual process that leads to long-lasting advantages.

Practical Tips for Transitioning

Transitioning to a diet focused on raw foods involves significant preparation and attention.

Here are some practical ways to make the process smoother:

1. Gradual Change: Rather than trying an abrupt overhaul of your diet, consider adopting modest, lasting improvements. Start by substituting one or two ultra-processed snacks or meals with whole-food alternatives each week.

2. *Label Scrutiny:* When shopping for groceries, pay great attention to food labels. Opt for products with few ingredients, and if feasible, pick foods without a label: fresh fruits, vegetables, and lean meats.

3. *Home Cooking:* Preparing your meals at home enables you to have greater control over the ingredients. Experiment with cooking and enjoy the creative process of producing your cuisine.

4. *Batch Cooking:* To save time and ensure you have unprocessed choices readily accessible, try batch cooking. Prepare bigger amounts of soups, stews, and cereals, and freeze portions for future meals.

5. *Snack Prep:* Have a range of healthy, unprocessed foods available. Snacking on fresh fruits, vegetables, nuts, and seeds might help avoid the temptation of processed alternatives.

6. Explore Farmer's Markets: Visiting local farmer's markets may be a lovely way to find fresh, uncooked food. It also helps local farmers and develops a sense of community.

Unprocessed food alternatives

Here's a list of some typical ultra-processed foods and their unprocessed alternatives:

1. Chips and Snack Bars: Instead of potato chips or sugary snack bars, seek out raw almonds, seeds, or air-popped popcorn. You may also build your own trail mix using a combination of nuts, dried fruits, and dark chocolate chunks.

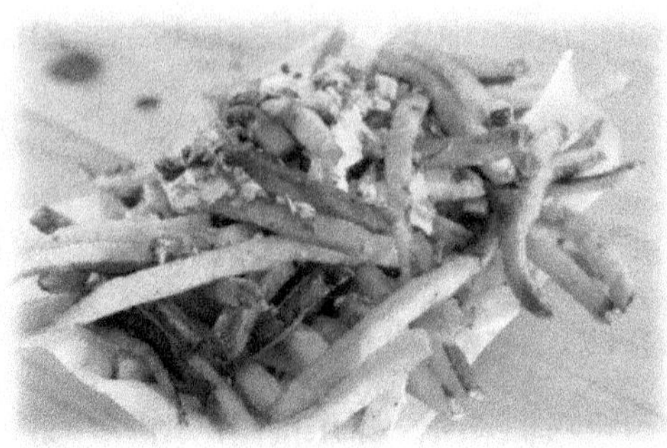

2. Soda and Sugary Drinks: Replace sugary sodas with sparkling water enriched with fresh fruit slices or unsweetened herbal tea. Water with a touch of lemon or lime is a wonderful alternative too.

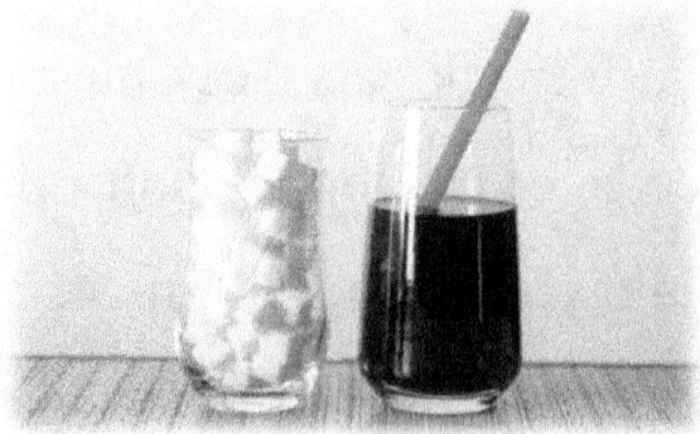

3. Canned Soups: Swap canned soups loaded with salt and additives for homemade soups prepared from fresh veggies, herbs, and lean meats. It's a healthy and soothing alternative.

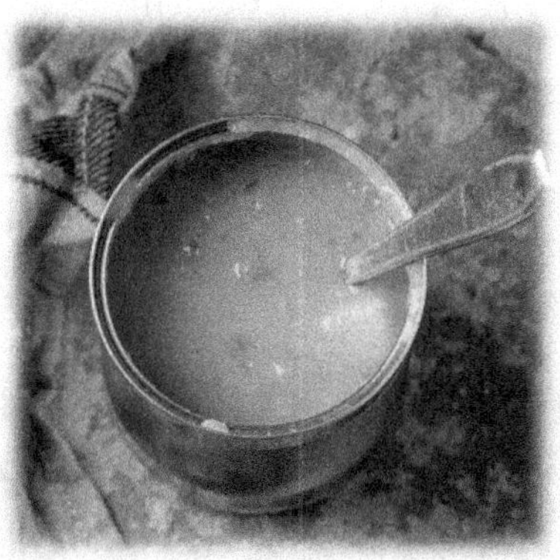

4. Frozen Dinners: Instead of frozen, processed dinners, produce your own frozen meals by batch cooking and freezing portions of your home-cooked foods. These will be free from additives and suited to your preferences.

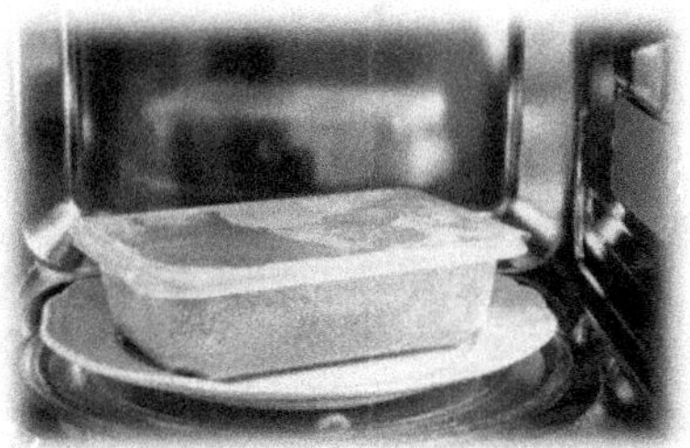

5. Candy and Sweets: Opt for natural sweetness by indulging in fresh, whole fruits like berries, apples, and citrus. Dark chocolate with a high cocoa content may also be a delicious treat.

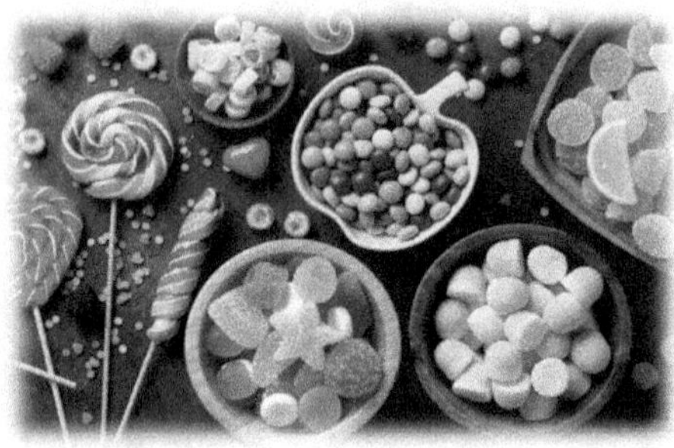

6. Processed Meats: Substitute processed deli meats with freshly roasted or grilled lean proteins, such as turkey or chicken breast. They may be used for sandwiches or salads.

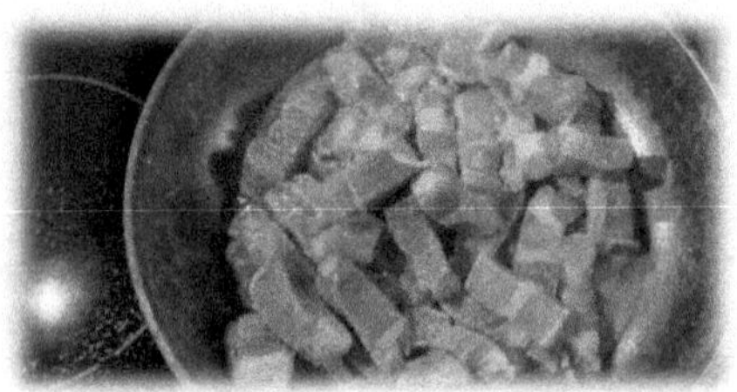

Unprocessed food recipes

To inspire your culinary journey towards unprocessed meals, here are a few dishes that include entire, unprocessed ingredients:

1. Grilled Vegetable Platter:

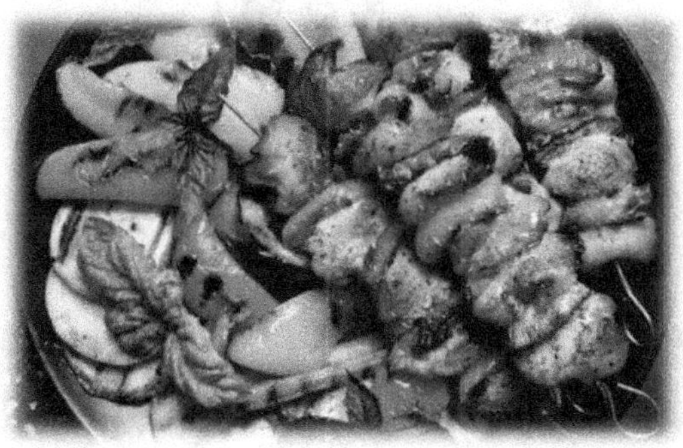

Ingredients: Fresh zucchini, bell peppers, eggplant, and cherry tomatoes.

Instructions: Slice the veggies and grill them with a sprinkle of olive oil, garlic, and herbs. Serve on a colorful plate with a side of hummus.

2. Quinoa and Black Bean Salad:

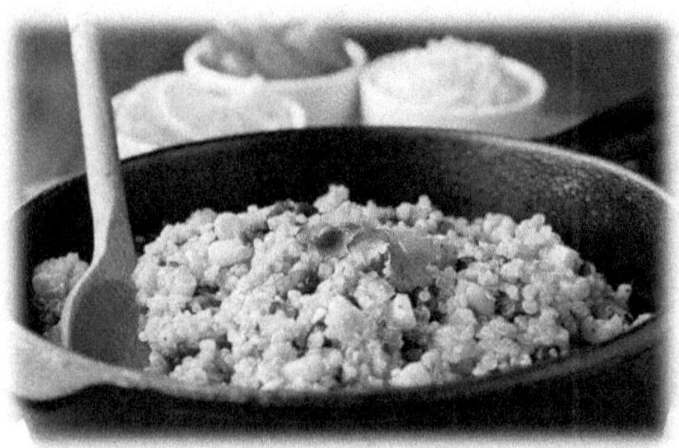

Ingredients: Quinoa, black beans, fresh corn, bell pepper, cilantro, and lime vinaigrette.

Instructions: Cook the quinoa and combine it with the beans, corn, diced pepper, and cilantro. Drizzle with the lime vinaigrette for a delicious salad.

3. Overnight Oats with Berries:

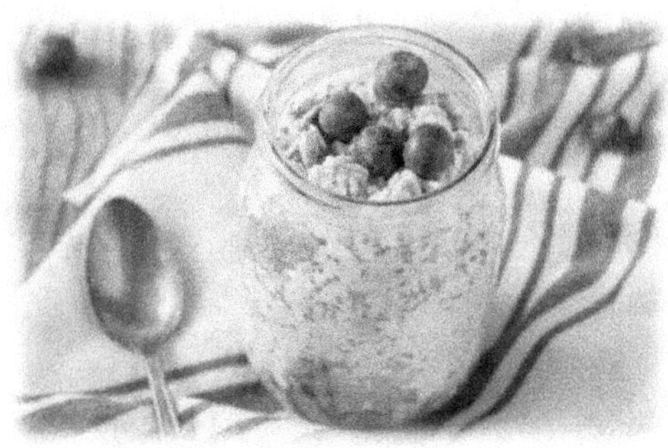

Ingredients: Rolled oats, Greek yogurt, fresh berries, honey, and chia seeds.

Instructions: Mix the oats, yogurt, chia seeds, and a sprinkle of honey in a container. Top with fresh berries and refrigerate overnight for a healthy breakfast.

4. Grilled Chicken with Lemon and Rosemary:

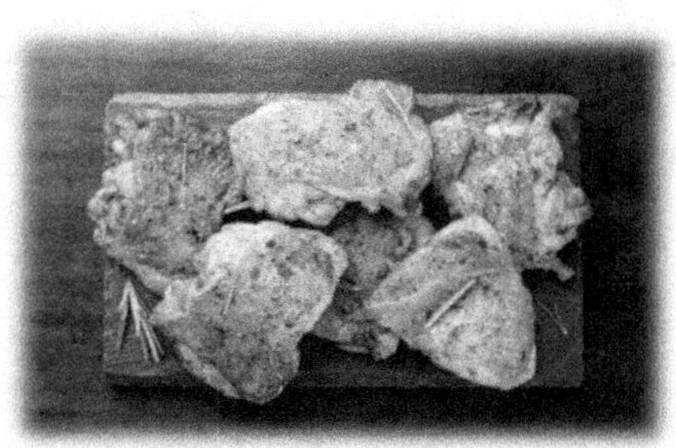

Ingredients: boneless chicken breasts, fresh rosemary, lemon juice, and garlic.

Instructions: Marinate the chicken in a combination of lemon juice, garlic, and fresh rosemary. Grill until thoroughly done and enjoy a tasty, unprocessed dinner.

5. Homemade Trail Mix:

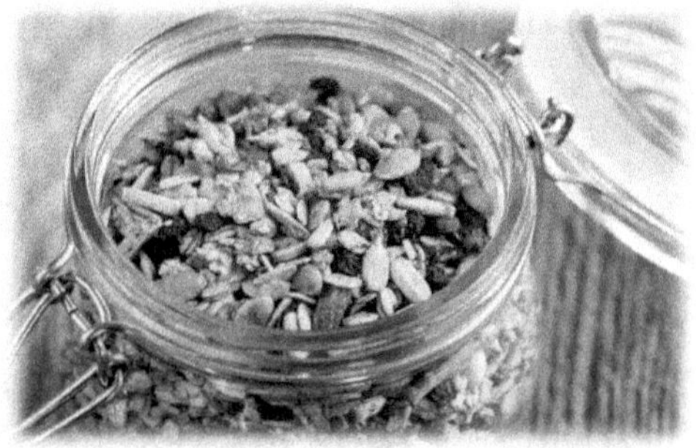

Ingredients: almonds, walnuts, dried cranberries, dark chocolate bits, and pumpkin seeds.

Instructions: Mix the items together to make your unique trail mix. It's a handy and healthy snack for on-the-go.

The journey continues.

Your path towards unprocessed foods is not simply a momentary shift; it's a step towards a healthier and more vibrant existence. This chapter serves as your guide to adopting practical strategies, finding unprocessed alternatives, and exploring delectable dishes. Remember, every healthy meal and snack you select is a step closer to a healthier you.

In the following chapter, we'll dig into the implications of bad eating and investigate how your food choices may affect numerous parts of your health, from stable blood pressure to skin cancer and diabetes.

CHAPTER 8

HEALTH CONSEQUENCES OF UNHEALTHY EATING

In this chapter, we start with a key investigation of the significant and frequently disturbing repercussions of bad eating habits, especially those related to the intake of ultra-processed foods. As we look into the possible implications of these dietary choices on many elements of health, it becomes clearly evident that our food choices profoundly affect our overall well-being.

The Complex Web of Health and Diet

Understanding the complicated link between eating choices and health consequences is vital.

Our bodies act as finely calibrated machines, and the fuel we offer them our food plays an indisputable role in determining how effectively they perform. It's not only about calories in vs. calories out; it's about the quality and mix of the calories we eat.

Blood Pressure and the Effects of Processed Foods

One of the direct repercussions of ingesting ultra-processed meals is the possible influence on blood pressure. These goods, generally heavy in salt, may lead to a rise in blood pressure levels, which, if uncontrolled, can contribute to diseases like hypertension. In turn, hypertension is a well-established risk factor for heart disease, stroke, and other cardiovascular disorders.

In a study published in the Journal of Hypertension, researchers noticed that those who consumed a diet high in ultra-processed foods had a considerably increased chance of developing high blood pressure compared to those who maintained a diet centered on whole, unprocessed foods. This research underlines the clear relationship between food choices and their repercussions on blood pressure.

The Connection between Allergies and Skin Health

While it may not be immediately evident, our food choices may also affect the development of allergies and skin health. The ingestion of highly processed meals may lead to a number of difficulties, including food allergies and intolerances. These diseases may appear with a range of symptoms, such as skin rashes, hives, and gastrointestinal problems.

It's worth mentioning that some chemicals and preservatives typically found in ultra-processed meals may intensify these responses. The inclusion of artificial colors, flavors, and preservatives has been connected with severe skin responses in certain people.

Chronic diseases and diet-induced health consequences

Perhaps the most worrying feature of bad eating habits is their influence on the development of chronic illnesses. This chapter covers in detail how our food choices might eventually lead to health conditions like type 2 diabetes.

Type 2 Diabetes: Research has repeatedly demonstrated that diets heavy in ultra-processed foods, typified by excessive sugar and harmful fats, may considerably raise the risk of type 2 diabetes. Research published in the Journal of Diabetes Care indicated that those who consumed a diet heavy in these processed items had a substantially greater probability of acquiring type 2 diabetes compared to those who opted for a diet focused on whole, unprocessed foods.

This worrying association underlines the significance of being careful with food choices, since the effects of bad eating habits may be severe. Through statistics, case stories, and scientific discoveries, we hope to shed light on the severe health repercussions that may emerge from bad diets.

A Multifaceted Approach to Health

It's crucial to remember that health is diverse, and the implications of improper eating habits may be both immediate and long-term. The impacts extend beyond simply the physical aspect, touching our emotional and mental well-being as well.

Emotional Well-being: Studies have demonstrated a correlation between the intake of ultra-processed meals and an increased risk of depression and anxiety. The nutrient-poor quality of these items may leave us feeling sluggish, angry, and even emotionally unstable.

Mental Health: The association between nutrition and mental health is an emerging subject of inquiry. A diet heavy in ultra-processed foods may have ties to cognitive decline and mental health issues. While it's a complicated subject, our food choices surely play a part in preserving brain clarity and general cognitive health.

Long-term Wellness: The development of chronic illnesses owing to improper eating habits frequently comes with long-term health management. Conditions including type 2 diabetes, hypertension, or skin allergies might need continual care, medicine, and lifestyle adjustments.

The Journey to a Healthier You

While this chapter digs into the depressing repercussions of poor eating, it's vital to remember that information is the first step towards change. The ultimate objective is to empower you with the understanding required to make educated food choices that emphasize your health and well-being. As we move through this book, we'll also discuss practical answers and tactics for making better choices. We will give advice on how to identify and limit the intake of ultra-processed foods, suggesting tangible strategies to create a more nutritious and balanced diet.

In the following chapter, we'll cover one of the most effective approaches to addressing the bad eating patterns linked with ultra-processed foods: understanding and applying no-processed food recipes. These dishes, rich in unprocessed foods, provide a tasty and healthy alternative to processed meals and snacks.

CHAPTER 9

NUTRITION FOR ACTIVE LIFESTYLES

In this chapter, we move our emphasis towards a critical area of nutrition catering to the nutritional demands of those with busy lives. Specifically, we'll study the dietary needs of people active in sports and high-intensity physical activity like cross-country running. The relevance of adequate nutrition cannot be overemphasized when it comes to increasing athletic performance, aiding recovery, and preserving general health.

Fueling the athlete within

cross-country running is a thrilling sport that demands stamina, endurance, and unflinching drive. The fuel that fuels this physical effort is, without a doubt, good nutrition. Athletes participating in such high-intensity sports have particular nutritional demands that vary from the normal person's diet.

The Importance of Calories

Active athletes, such as cross-country runners, expend a substantial quantity of calories throughout their training and competitions. It's vital to fulfill these higher energy needs to support both performance and recuperation. In this part, we'll go into the intricacies of caloric intake for athletes, underscoring the need to fuel the body sufficiently.

We'll also explore the idea of a "caloric deficit" vs. a "caloric surplus" and how these variables might impact athletic performance. Through case stories and scientific results, we'll highlight the real advantages of feeding the body with the energy it needs.

Staying Hydrated: A Non-Negotiable Requirement

Cross-country running generally takes place in a range of locales and weather situations, which may contribute to significant fluid loss via perspiration. Dehydration may have adverse impacts on an athlete's performance and health. We'll review the repercussions of dehydration and underline the crucial need to keep hydrated.

In addition to recognizing the significance of hydration, we'll share practical recommendations on fluid consumption before, during, and after training and events. By merging scientific insights and real-life athlete experiences, we want to underline the relevance of optimal hydration to sports achievement.

Nutrient Optimization for Athletic Performance

The cross-country runner's diet should go beyond merely fulfilling caloric demands and water. The diet should also concentrate on optimizing nutrition intake to boost sports performance. Here, we'll review the relevance of several nutrients and how they impact endurance, muscle repair, and general well-being.

Carbohydrates: Carbohydrates are the major source of energy for endurance athletes. We'll investigate how the body stores and utilizes carbs throughout lengthy periods of activity. Additionally, we'll give information on carbohydrate loading tactics and the need for balanced carbohydrate consumption.

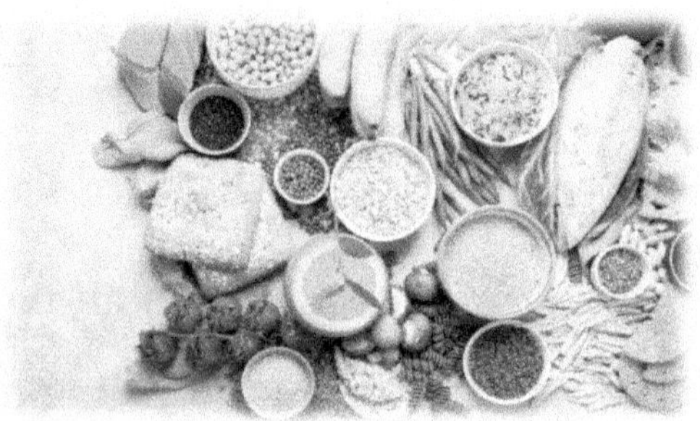

Proteins: The importance of proteins in muscle repair and recovery is well known. Cross-country runners, like other athletes, must maintain a protein-rich diet to sustain their training efforts. We'll look into the science behind protein's significance in endurance sports and give guidance on protein-rich dietary choices.

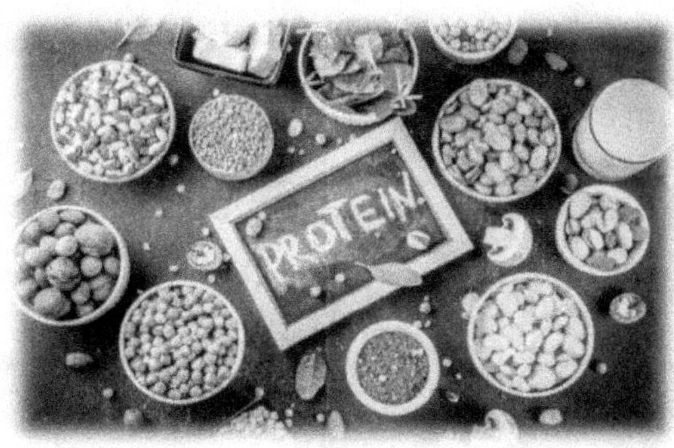

Fats: Dietary fats are a vital energy source, especially during longer endurance exercises. We'll study the role of fats in energy generation and give insights into the sorts of fats that are most advantageous for athletes.

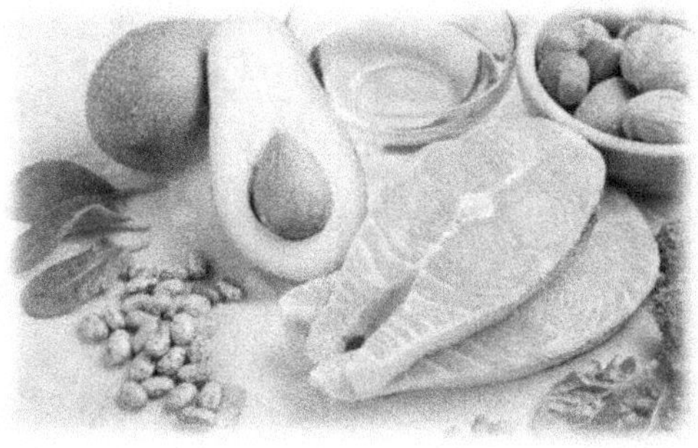

Micronutrients: Beyond macronutrients like carbs, proteins, and fats, we'll cover the value of micronutrients such as vitamins and minerals. These micronutrients play a key role in activities including oxygen transfer, muscular contraction, and immunological maintenance. We'll provide assistance in reaching these micronutrient demands through food choices.

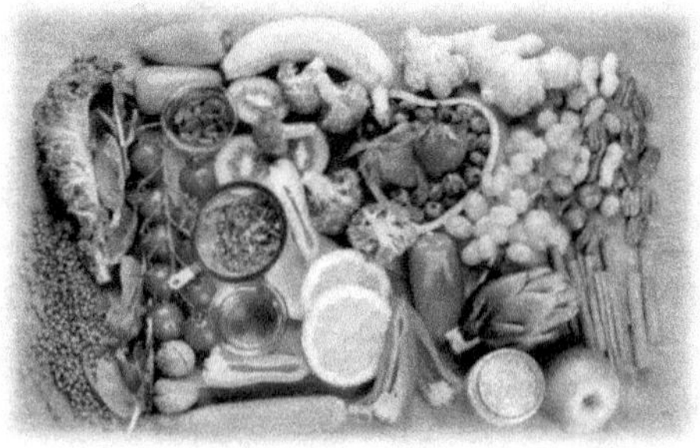

Nutrition and athletic excellence

This chapter stresses the crucial role that nutrition plays in the lives of active humans, particularly cross-country runners. We want to provide athletes with the information and insights required to make intelligent food decisions that will enhance their performance, help recovery, and preserve their general health. By offering a complete grasp of the dietary needs of people with active lives, we strive to promote the athletic interests of readers. In the following chapter, we'll delve deeper into the realm of nutrition, studying the value of a balanced and varied diet and the particular foods that may power an active lifestyle.

CHAPTER 10

IDENTIFYING AND AVOIDING ULTRA-PROCESSED FOODS

In this last chapter, we'll give readers practical ways for recognizing and, more importantly, avoiding ultra-processed meals. Armed with the information you've received from earlier chapters, you're now better positioned to make educated decisions about the food you eat. We'll go into the art of reading food labels, detecting hidden chemicals and ingredients, and giving vital ideas for avoiding ultra-processed meals while embracing natural, unprocessed alternatives.

Navigating the supermarket aisles

The normal store is a maze of possibilities, where ultra-processed goods frequently lurk around every corner. This section is meant to be your guide, helping you traverse these aisles with confidence and understanding.

Understanding food labels

Food labels may be complicated, and it's easy to be deceived by marketing practices. We'll present you with step-by-step guidance on interpreting food labels. Learn to recognize key information like serving sizes, nutritional content, and ingredient lists. With this talent, you can make educated decisions and better grasp what's within the packaged meals you're contemplating.

Recognizing Hidden Additives

Many ultra-processed foods are packed with chemicals and preservatives, frequently masked beneath obscure labels. This section sheds light on common additives, enabling you to spot them on labels. Armed with this information, you may spot those meals and beverages that may not be as healthy as they appear.

Tips for Avoiding Ultra-Processed Foods

Eradicating ultra-processed foods from your diet may seem like a big endeavor, particularly if they've been mainstays in your life for years. We'll present a series of practical, concrete ideas for progressively phasing out these items and adopting a diet focused on complete, unadulterated alternatives.

Building a healthier plate

In this part, we'll examine the principles of designing a healthy plate, beginning with a balanced and diverse diet.

The Balanced Plate: Creating a balanced plate is about ensuring that your food is diversified, providing a broad assortment of critical nutrients. We'll discuss what a balanced plate looks like, stressing the necessity of including items from all food categories. By the conclusion of this part, you'll have a better concept of what a healthy lunch should consist of.

Whole, unprocessed alternatives: Embracing complete, unprocessed alternatives is a cornerstone of better eating. We'll offer you a thorough list of whole foods that can substitute for their ultra-processed competitors. For instance, if you're used to sugary morning cereals, we'll propose healthy choices like whole grains, oats, and fresh fruits.

Cooking and meal preparation

This section focuses on the practical side of adding whole, unprocessed foods to your everyday meals. We'll explore techniques for meal planning, preparation, and cooking.

Meal Planning: Meal planning is a vital step in shifting to a diet centered on healthy foods. We'll share insights into efficient meal planning, including ideas on developing balanced and healthy meal plans, which foods to prioritize, and how to guarantee that you have access to fresh products.

Meal Preparation: To support a lifestyle centered on nutritious foods, meal planning may be a game-changer. This section gives tips on how to make meal preparation a part of your routine. We'll cover the fundamentals of meal planning, from picking the correct containers to keeping cooked meals secure.

Cooking with Whole Foods

Cooking with whole foods may be a fun and gratifying experience. In this segment, we'll examine how to cook healthy and tasty meals utilizing whole, unprocessed products. We'll present a variety of easy-to-follow recipes to help you get started on your road towards healthy eating.

A Journey Towards Healthier Eating

In the last half of this chapter, we'll underline the need for gradual transformation. Transitioning from an ultra-processed diet to one centered on whole foods is a huge transition. We'll provide advice on pacing yourself and maintaining consistency. You'll discover suggestions on keeping motivated and adopting a sustainable approach to eating healthily.

In Conclusion: In this chapter, you've begun the adventure of finding and rejecting ultra-processed foods while embracing complete, unprocessed alternatives. By learning the art of reading food labels and spotting hidden substances, you've earned the abilities required to make educated decisions about what you eat.

As you continue your road towards healthy eating, you'll be more able to navigate the grocery aisles, construct a healthier plate, and increase your meal preparation abilities. The objective is not simply to avoid ultra-processed foods but also to relish in the advantages of a diet that values full, unprocessed foodstuffs.

In the last chapter, we'll reflect on the entire adventure you've undertaken. We'll highlight the important insights from this book and leave you with a motivational message, reiterating the merits of adopting full, unprocessed foods in your diet.

CONCLUSION

As we approach the close of our voyage into the world of ultra-processed foods and the hunt for healthy eating habits, it's time to reflect on the major points from each chapter. We've gone on a journey to investigate the effect of ultra-processed foods on our diets and health. We've explored the science behind these foods, the hidden risks lying therein, and the nutritional repercussions of ingesting them. We've investigated the role of genetics in affecting our reaction to varied diets and identified the road to avoiding ultra-processed meals while embracing complete, unprocessed alternatives.

A Recap of the Journey

Understanding Ultra-Processed Foods: We started by defining what ultra-processed foods are and separating them from their less-processed alternatives. We've learned to identify these items, both from their ingredient labels and their presence on the grocery shelves.

The Science Behind Ultra-Processed Foods: In the second chapter, we dug into the complicated science of food processing, dissecting the mechanisms that make ultra-processed foodstuffs. We studied the function of different ingredients and additives in boosting taste, texture, and shelf life.

The Hidden Dangers: Ingredients and additives: We uncovered the possible health concerns connected with common chemicals and preservatives in ultra-processed meals. Armed with this information, you may now recognize and comprehend the effects of taking these components.

Nutrition and Ultra-Processed Foods: The fourth chapter compared the nutritional value of ultra-processed foods to whole, unprocessed meals. We've covered the possible nutritional effects of reliance on ultra-processed meals, including the possibility of vitamin shortages.

Genetics and Weight: Exploring the Connection We've investigated the interesting impact of genetics on influencing an individual's weight and body composition. Our quest via genetics demonstrated how various diets and food kinds may interact with our particular genetic composition.

Unprocessed Food Alternatives: In the sixth chapter, we've given you the skills to shift to a diet focused on unprocessed foods. From practical tips to particular examples and a range of recipes, you're now well-equipped to explore entire, unprocessed foods.

Health repercussions of bad eating habits: We've covered the health repercussions of bad eating habits, throwing light on the possible impacts on blood pressure, allergies, skin health, and the development of chronic illnesses like type 2 diabetes. The relationship between ultra-processed meals and these health effects is obvious today.

Nutrition for Active Lifestyles: For individuals living active lifestyles, we've looked into the dietary needs to promote sports performance, rehabilitation, and general well-being. A proper diet may boost your physical skills and help you fulfill the demands of an active lifestyle.

Identifying and Avoiding Ultra-Processed Foods: This last chapter is your guide to identifying and avoiding ultra-processed foods. By learning the skill of reading food labels, spotting hidden ingredients, and adopting practical advice, you're better able to make educated decisions about the food you eat.

Taking Action and Embracing Change: As you've gone through this book, you've gathered a lot of information about the foods you consume and their possible influence on your health. It's now time to take action and make educated decisions regarding your nutrition. A route to healthy eating habits is one that may need change, and change is frequently easier when it's gradual.

Remember that tiny, persistent actions may lead to major changes in your overall well-being. Start by evaluating your personal diet and finding areas where you may limit your use of ultra-processed foods. Embrace full, unprocessed alternatives and experiment with cooking and food preparation. Gradually, you'll discover that better eating becomes a part of your routine.

A Motivating Message of Hope: In closing, I want to leave you with a message of optimism. Adopting healthy eating habits may have a tremendous influence on your life. It's not only about the absence of ultra-processed meals but also about the availability of nutrient-rich, complete components that may feed your body and nurture your well-being. The road towards healthy eating is one of self-discovery, empowerment, and energy.

By making educated decisions about your diet and selecting whole, unadulterated foods, you're taking a huge step towards a healthier, happier self. Improved well-being, improved energy, and a decreased risk of chronic illnesses are just some of the pleasures awaiting you on this road. Remember, you have the ability to mold your food choices, and in doing so, you're creating your future. Embrace this journey to improved eating habits with confidence and excitement. Your body and your health will reward you for it.